THE LITTLE BOOK OF
BACH FLOWER REMEDIES

THE LITTLE BOOK OF

BACH FLOWER REMEDIES

Practical tips for effective
self-treatment

SVEN SOMMER

Vermilion
LONDON

5 7 9 10 8 6

First published in 2002 by Vermilion,
an imprint of Ebury Publishing

A Random House Group company

The Random House Group Limited Reg. No. 954009

Addresses for companies within the Random House Group can be found at:
www.randomhouse.co.uk

A CIP catalogue record for this book is available from the British Library

The Random House Group Limited supports The Forest Stewardship Council
(FSC), the leading international forest certification organisation. All our titles th
are printed on Greenpeace approved FSC certified paper carry the FSC logo.
Our paper procurement policy can be found at:
www.randomhouse.co.uk/environment

Printed and bound in China

ISBN 9780091884291

Copies are available at special rates for bulk orders. Contact the sales
development team on 020 7840 8487 for more information.

To buy books by your favourite authors
and register for offers, visit
www.randomhouse.co.uk

CONTENTS

For my parents

I want to thank Claudia Herbert, clinical psychologist and director of the Oxford Development Centre Ltd, for her valuable advice.

The information in this book is intended to be advisory in nature and should not be regarded as a replacement for professional medical or psychological treatment or advice. If in doubt, always consult your GP, psychologist/psychotherapist or an experienced practitioner. Neither the publishers nor the author of this book can be held liable for any errors, omissions or actions that may be taken as a consequence of using it.

DEAR READER

Welcome to THE LITTLE BOOK OF BACH FLOWER REMEDIES, a concise but comprehensive introduction to the world of healing with Bach Remedies.

In my own practice I often use Bach Remedies in conjunction with other complementary therapies such as homeopathy, acupuncture or naturopathy. With this book you can experience firsthand a gentle but effective way of healing. Free from any side-effects, Bach Remedies are perfectly suited to self-treatment for emotional conditions as well as physical complaints.

Sven Sommer

PART ONE

WHAT ARE BACH REMEDIES?

Bach Remedies were discovered by Dr Edward Bach (1886–1936). Dissatisfied with the results of conventional medicine he initially turned to homeopathy in the hope of finding a better alternative. He came to believe that each of us is by nature happy and healthy, as long as we are in touch with our inner self. It is when we lose this harmonious connection with our inner being that negative emotions, such as fear, uncertainty, anger or desperation, arise. Bach believed that these emotional imbalances were the real reason behind any illness or distress.

In the 1930s, Bach discovered the first plants which had a healing effect on negative states of mind. In his research he identified a total of 38 plants which can be used to treat a variety of negative emotional states. For the most part, Bach used the flowers of these wild growing plants to prepare his remedies or essences. This is why their full title is the Bach Flower Remedies.

For Edward Bach it was essential to keep his system of healing safe and simple. He hoped that one day every household would use it. Today we are becoming increasingly attuned to our emotional well-being and how closely this relates to our physical health. Self-treatment with Bach Remedies may become an essential part of our modern lifestyle.

RESCUE REMEDY

Bach's *Rescue Remedy* is a ready-made mixture of five Bach Remedies (*Cherry Plum, Clematis, Impatiens, Rock Rose* and *Star of Bethlehem*). This mixture was created by Dr Bach himself, who claimed to have saved lives with it. It is by far the most well known of the Bach Remedies.

Rescue Remedy is extremely useful whenever you feel completely overwhelmed and for every kind of emergency – for unconsciousness or fainting, acute fears, panic attacks, and whenever your body, mind or soul has received a shock or is in great distress. This might be a psychological shock caused, for example, by a burglary, a physical shock from an accident (e.g. cuts, burns, strains) or an operation, a mental shock such as the loss of a loved one, or one of the many daily 'small' shocks, such as being shouted at by someone at work. *Rescue Remedy* will help you to regain your inner equilibrium and its calming effect often takes hold within minutes. It is also highly recommended for treating children.

For all smaller shocks and accidents a couple of drops or some of the cream can work miracles. Put 2–3 drops directly on the tongue (or lips) or 3 drops in a small glass of water or other liquid and sip at intervals until you feel some improvement. For external use, in cases of strains, slight burns, tensions and skin problems, dilute 12 drops in half a litre (1 pint) of water and use it as a compress.

Bach Rescue Cream has healing, soothing properties which can help with a wide variety of skin conditions such as rough or flaking skin. Repeat application whenever needed.

Please note that in all emergencies First Aid must take priority! Only then should *Rescue Remedy* be used if appropriate. I highly recommend having a bottle of *Rescue Remedy* drops at home, at work and whenever you are travelling.

HEAL YOURSELF – WHEN TO USE BACH REMEDIES

Heal Thyself was the title of one of Bach's publications. It was very important to him that his method was easy to understand and very easy to use, so that everyone could benefit from it.

1. Emotional problems

This is the real strength of treatment with Bach Remedies. Bach saw that emotional imbalances could lead to distress, which affects our vitality and can subsequently make us ill. If you suffer from negative emotions, such as anger problems, impatience, jealousy or envy, Bach Remedies can help you to regain your inner balance and prevent illness.

2. Strengthening your inner balance and helping with personal development

If you are by nature shy or suffer from uncertainty or a lack of self-confidence, if you feel easily anxious or depressed, if your children have learning problems or a fear of examinations, Bach Remedies can help to provide inner strength.

3. Treatment of illness

Dr Bach recognized that the same disease may have different effects on different people – while one patient may become very anxious, another may become withdrawn. Bach believed that the differing emotions themselves should be treated. In chronic conditions the sufferer often becomes more irritable, bitter or aggressive. Bach Remedies can help with these negative states of mind and can therefore give new hope and peace of mind. Even people with a terminal illness may find comfort and relief from them.

4 . For shocks and in emergencies
Rescue Remedy, a mixture of five different Bach Remedies, has become well known as a treatment for all kinds of emotional and physical shocks and other emergencies. (For more details see page 14.)

Which Bach Remedies to choose depends on your state of mind. Look out for negative emotional states, a negative approach or perspective on life, negative behaviour and negative interactions with other people.

Begin with your present problem. You can then go on to peel away further negative emotional layers, one by one. Bach Remedies will help you to win back your inner harmony and balance, and in so doing help to heal your body and your soul.

HOW TO FIND THE RIGHT BACH REMEDIES

1. To find the right remedies ask yourself:
   - What do I feel at the moment?
     (e.g. desperate, fearful, insecure,
     tired)
   - How do I behave at the moment?
     (e.g. am I being intolerant, aggressive,
     panicky?)
   - How do I feel generally? (e.g. shy,
     lacking self-confidence, depressed)
   - How do I behave generally? (e.g. am I
     being bitter, impatient, jealous, with-
     drawn?)
2. The questionnaire that follows will help
   you to establish how you feel and give
   you some first indications as to which
   remedies might be suitable.

3. If you have an emotional problem or physical complaint read the brief descriptions of the remedies on pages 34–81.

4. Choose the remedies which best match your condition. You can choose up to seven Bach Remedies to create your own individual mixture (see also page 182 The Way to Take Bach Remedies).

If you find more than seven Bach Remedies, concentrate on those which best correspond to your acute problems (see under point 1 on page 21). These are usually fewer than seven. You can then add one or two Remedies for the longer lasting problems or physical complaints. If none of the descriptions match your symptoms you cannot help yourself with this book. If this is the case you should consult a trained Bach practitioner.

THE QUESTIONNAIRE

This small questionnaire will help you to select the Bach Remedies most suitable for you. Try to answer the questions spontaneously.

Tick box A if the question correlates to one of your more acute emotional problems at the moment.

Tick box C if the question correlates to one of your more long-term or chronic emotional problems.

If you tick more than seven questions go through the questionnaire again and grade the questions you have ticked (1 for mild, 2 for medium, 3 for serious problems).

The number at the end of each question indicates the appropriate Bach Remedy. To find out which one it is refer to the list at the end of the questionnaire.

Consider taking the remedies you have ticked or, if you chose more than seven remedies, which have the highest scores.

	A	C
• Do you hide your worries, fears, anxieties and restlessness behind humour and a brave face? (1)		
• Do you have a tendency to avoid thinking about your problems (e.g. through drugs, alcohol, seeking distraction)? (1)		
• Do you suffer from unexplained fears, worries, anxieties or apprehension? (2)		
• Do you easily feel intolerant of others or their behaviour? (3)		
• Do you have problems saying 'no' to other people's needs or demands? (4)		

- Do you ask frequently for advice, because you do not trust your own judgement? (5)

- Do you have uncontrolled irrational thoughts or a fear of losing control? (6)

- Do you keep repeating the same mistakes and seem unable to learn from experience? (7)

- Do you feel hurt, neglected or unloved by some friend or family member? (8)

- Do you feel rather possessive about some loved ones, and that you cannot let them go? (8)

- Do you tend to be indifferent, absent-minded, a day-dreamer, or do you try to escape from reality? (9)

- Do you have an excessive need for order – to clean, to wash or to tidy up? (10)

- Do you feel unclean, infected, or suffer from self-disgust? (10)

- Do you feel temporarily desperate, stressed, overwhelmed or exhausted by responsibilities? (11)

- Do you feel discouraged, doubtful, pessimistic and sceptical (perhaps because you've suffered a set-back)? (12)

- Have you given up all hope and do you feel lost? (13)

- Do you dwell on the past? (16)

- Are you preoccupied with your own problems? (14)

A | C

- Do you experience negative and destructive thoughts (such as hate, rage, jealousy or envy? (15)
- Do you feel tired, floppy and unmotivated? (17)
- Do you get impatient easily? (18)
- Do you lack self-confidence and have a tendency to feel inferior? (19)
- Do you suffer from any specific fears or phobias? (20)
- Do you feel depressed or melancholic without reason? (21)
- Have you pushed yourself too hard, without admitting it to yourself or others? (22)
- Do you feel exhausted and weak? (23)
- Are you timid and shy? (20)

A | C

- Do you feel guilty about something you have done or left undone? (24)

- Do you feel responsible for the faults or mistakes of others? (24)

- Do you worry obsessively about others? (25)

- Do you experience acute terror, panic and fear? (26)

- Do you strive for perfectionism and push yourself to achieve high goals? (27)

- Are you strict with yourself, denying yourself pleasure or joy in life? (17)

- Do you suffer from mood swings? (28)

- Do you have problems deciding between two options? (28)

- Have you experienced some shock or trauma from which you have not yet recovered? (29)

- Do you feel deep anguish and despair, and at the limits of your endurance? (30)

- Do you feel stressed, tense or worn out, because you are over-enthusiastic about certain ideas or projects? (31)

- Do you have a tendency to control other people, to be inflexible and unable to tolerate contradiction? (32)

- Are you over-sensitive to external influences? (33)

- Are you struggling to adapt to a new situation in your life? (33)

- Do you have a tendency to withdraw and be on your own? (34)

- Do you prefer not to bother other people with your problems? (34)

- Do you have persistent, repetitive and unwanted thoughts? (35)

- Do you have many ideas and plans, but are indecisive about what to do? (36)

- Do you feel frustrated, because you have not yet found your purpose in life? (36)

- Do you suffer from a lack of vitality? (37)

- Have you submitted to your fate, and so feel apathetic? (37)

- Do you feel bitter, resentful or unfairly treated? (38)

The number at the end of each question represents a Bach Remedy:

(1) Agrimony, (2) Aspen, (3) Beech, (4) Centaury, (5) Cerato, (6) Cherry Plum, (7) Chestnut Bud, (8) Chicory, (9) Clematis, (10) Crab Apple, (11) Elm, (12) Gentian, (13) Gorse, (14) Heather, (15) Holly, (16) Honeysuckle, (17) Hornbeam, (18) Impatiens, (19) Larch, (20) Mimulus, (21) Mustard, (22) Oak, (23) Olive, (24) Pine, (25) Red Chestnut, (26) Rock Rose, (27) Rock Water, (28) Scleranthus, (29) Star of Bethlehem, (30) Sweet Chestnut, (31) Vervain, (32) Vine, (33) Walnut, (34) Water Violet, (35) White Chestnut, (36) Wild Oat, (37) Wild Rose, (38) Willow

PART
TWO

THE COMPLETE REMEDIES
FROM A TO Z

In this chapter you will find a brief introduction to each of the 38 Bach Remedies
mentioned in this book. Under each
remedy you will find a brief description of
the complaints and conditions known to
respond well to that particular remedy.
This is followed by a list of the main associated emotional and physical symptoms.
This information should help you to make
your choice, especially if you have difficulty
in deciding between several different
remedies.

(1) Agrimony

Agrimonia eupatoria

For hidden anxiety

Recommended for those who hide their fears, worries and restlessness behind humour and a 'brave face'.

Main symptoms:
- cheerful, humorous, seek harmony, avoid arguments, adopt a 'keep smiling' policy
- seek out company of others, to avoid being alone
- take alcohol or drugs to dull their pain
- avoid showing or talking about their feelings
- internal restlessness
- find it hard to concentrate

Physical symptoms:
- addictions, nervousness, restlessness,

insomnia, grinding teeth, nail biting, nervous skin irritations

(2) Aspen

Populus tremula

For anxiety and unknown fears

Recommended for those who suffer from unknown fears and apprehension.

Main symptoms:
- a general, vague feeling of fear or danger with no reason or explanation; afraid to talk about it
- superstitious, fear of ghosts, dying, the dark; fear of spiders or snakes, of being punished, of being followed, etc.
- nightmares, cannot get back to sleep
- a general feeling of anxiety regarding certain places, people or situations

- withdrawal symptoms from alcohol or drugs, after-effects of drugs, post-traumatic stress

Possible physical symptoms:
- panic with trembling, perspiration, fainting

(3) Beech

Fagus sylvatica

For intolerance

Recommended for people who tend to be arrogant, critical and intolerant of others.

Main symptoms:
- dogmatic and pedantic behaviour
- constantly notice other people's mistakes; judgemental
- self-righteous – cannot accept any opinion other than their own

- impatient and unable to keep an open mind
- easily irritated by other people's habits and behaviour

Possible physical symptoms:
- stiffness, tension, irritability, digestive and absorption problems, allergic to hair, pollen, certain foods, etc.

(4) Centaury

Centaurium umbellatum

For submissiveness

Recommended for those who are weak-willed, easily exploited or imposed upon.

Main symptoms:
- easily dominated or bullied by others (e.g. partner, parent, boss), servile

- neglect their own needs in order to fulfil someone else's wishes
- lack of self-confidence – easily influenced by others, passive, shy
- give too much of themselves (time, energy …)
- very helpful to others, even servile
- cannot say 'no'; worry about hurting other people

Possible physical symptoms:
- tiredness, paleness (anaemia), lack of energy, backache, weak spine

(5) Cerato

Ceratostigma willmottiana

For distrusting yourself

Recommended for those who do not trust their own judgement and decisions.

Main symptoms:
- do not trust their own opinion or gut feelings
- constantly ask others for advice
- talk a lot, annoy others with questions
- cannot make spontaneous decisions
- try to give of their best, but feel insecure
- lack self-confidence, constantly changing their mind, self-doubting, easily influenced and manipulated by others
- dependent on someone else's opinion

Possible physical symptoms:
- nervous conditions, exhaustion

(6) Cherry Plum

Prunus cerasifera

For fear of losing control

Recommended for those who have uncontrolled, irrational thoughts.

Main symptoms:

- feel emotionally extremely 'blocked'
- fear of losing control, having a nervous breakdown, going mad
- fear of harming themselves or others; extreme desperation, thoughts of suicide; paranoia
- exploding, uncontrolled emotions, such as rage, hysteria, violence, aggression
- fear of releasing their emotions

Possible physical symptoms:

- very tense, restlessness, stuttering, bed-wetting, nail biting; useful during drug rehabilitation

(7) Chestnut Bud

Aesculus hippocastanum

For repeating mistakes

Recommended for those who make the same mistakes over and over again, who do not learn from experience.

Main symptoms:
- repeat the same mistakes in life, or at school, etc. because of lack of interest; find it difficult to learn or to concentrate
- easily lose things, easily confused, scatty and absent-minded
- restless and hasty; do not take time to learn from experience
- do not learn from the experience of others
- suffer from learning difficulties

Possible physical symptoms:
- periodically reappearing health problems such as stomach ulcers, migraine, acne, etc.

(8) Chicory

Chichorium intybus

For possessiveness

Recommended for those who are pre-occupied with their loved ones' well-being, are demanding, interfering and manipulative.

Main symptoms:
- over-caring; dominating; always know what is best for other people, constantly criticizing or commenting on others
- selfish and self-preoccupied; feel easily angry and resentful

- use emotional blackmail, demand constant sympathy, time and attention of others, become ill in order to get attention
- self-pity, feel easily hurt, neglected, unloved; play on their own unhappiness

Possible physical symptoms:
- eating disorders, liver and pancreas problems, diabetes, detox problems, constipation

(9) Clematis

Clematis vitalba

For dreaminess

Recommended for those who are absent-minded, day-dreamers, inattentive.

Main symptoms:
- avoid problems by withdrawing into a world of their own
- cannot concentrate, easily confused, sleepy, indifferent; often bump into things
- if ill, make little effort to recover; may even welcome the prospect of death
- escape from reality (by dreaming, playing computer games, watching TV, taking alcohol or drugs)

Possible physical symptoms:
- a lack of vitality or energy, tired, pale, fainting and loss of consciousness, cold hands and feet, sterility, hearing problems, problems with vision

(10) Crab Apple

Malus pumila

For cleansing

Recommended for those who feel unclean, infected, self-disgust and shame. Helps to detox.

Main symptoms:
- feel physically unclean, self-disgust caused by eczema, warts, acne, etc.; excessive need to tidy up, to wash, to clean themselves and/or their environment
- feel mentally unclean, self-disgust in relation to 'dirty' thoughts, fantasies, 'sins'
- fear contamination, illness, infection, pollution
- quickly feel desperate if treatment fails
- cannot accept own body or bodily functions (kissing, breast-feeding, passing stools)

Possible physical symptoms:
- skin problems (acne, eczema), flu, hangover, travel constipation

(11) Elm

Ulmus procera

For being overwhelmed and stressed

Recommended for those who are depressed, stressed or overwhelmed by responsibilities.

Main symptoms:
- very stressed and irritable
- feel suddenly overburdened, exhausted and despondent
- acute stress and burden cause desperation
- have taken too many things on board,

do not know where to start and how to cope
- strong characters who suddenly lack confidence or get depressed
- fear of breaking down

Possible physical symptoms:
- acute exhaustion, nervous breakdown, tension, insomnia, irritability, colds, sore throat, acute illness

(12) Gentian

Gentiana amarella

For discouragement

Recommended for those who are sceptical, doubtful and easily discouraged.

Main symptoms:
- feel depressed and know why

- have a sceptical, even pessimistic outlook on life
- lack will-power, feel disheartened even in the face of small obstacles
- give up easily and feel insecure because of a lack of self-confidence or faith
- discouraged by minor setbacks or failures
- always expect the worst

Possible physical symptoms:
- experience set-backs in the healing process, tendency to have recurring health problems

(13) Gorse

Ulex europaeus

For hopelessness

Recommended for those who have given up hope, feel defeated.

Main symptoms:
- feel too tired and depressed to change things for the better
- have given up – do not think anyone or anything can help
- feel defeated and deeply depressed after something has gone wrong
- might be convinced by friends and family to try various things, but deep inside feel pessimistic and beyond help
- despair

Possible physical symptoms:
- 'incurable' diseases, chronic illness

(14) Heather

Calluna vulgaris

For self-obsession

Recommended for people who are

obsessed with their own problems and talk constantly about themselves.

Main symptoms:
- cannot be alone, need an audience to talk to, to listen to their experiences, even though others get bored
- talkative, need to be the centre of attention
- only focused on their own problems, bad listener
- tend to be selfish, 'the needy child'
- try to impress others, inferiority complex
- suffer from results of past hurt or humiliation

Possible physical symptoms:
- digestive problems

(15) Holly

Ilex aquifolium

For negative and destructive thoughts

Recommended for those who have negative emotions such as anger, hatred, jealousy, suspicion, hostility, envy or resentment.

Main symptoms:
- easily unhappy, frustrated, without knowing why
- easily hurt
- given to attacks of anger, jealousy, etc.
- easily suspicious, suspect others of wrong doing
- choleric, aggressive even violent behaviour

Possible physical symptoms:
- illness with aggressive symptoms, such as high fever, severe inflammation or allergic reactions – all diseases and complaints which start with, or later develop, anger problems or irritability

(16) Honeysuckle

Lonicera caprifolium

For nostalgia

Recommended for those who are living in the past or feel homesick.

Main symptoms:
- tendency to neglect life in the present and to constantly dwell on the past
- glorify the past, everything was better then
- yearn for something (e.g. a lost dear

friend or home); tendency to brood
- tendency to bear a grudge, to be absent-minded; unable to concentrate
- nostalgic or homesick; do not accept anything new
- bad short-term but good long-term memory

Possible physical symptoms:
- deafness; problems with vision

(17) Hornbeam

Carpinus betulus

For physical and mental fatigue

Recommended for those who feel tired, 'floppy' and exhausted.

Main symptoms:
- feel more tired in the morning than in the evening
- feel weary, heavy headed and lacking in energy
- need coffee, tea or tonics to keep going
- do not think they can manage the tasks of the day, but feel better once they get going
- Monday-morning blues, hang-over feeling, (which clears up during the day); tired of the same job, of the same situation

Possible physical symptoms:
- low blood pressure, circulatory problems, tired eyes, fatigue, bad posture, short-sightedness, deafness

(18) Impatiens

Impatiens glandulifera

For impatience

Recommended for those who are easily impatient and irritated.

Main symptoms:
- nervous and easily irritated, restless; short-tempered and undiplomatic with others who slow them down

- everything has to happen at once, without delay – prefer to work alone, because others are not fast enough; tension and frustration because things happen too slowly (e.g. getting well)

- talk and think quickly, cannot sit still – have to be doing something constantly, tendency to overwork and exhaust themselves

Possible physical symptoms:
- nervous and restless, hyperactive, thyroid dysfunction, tics, spasms, insomnia, tension, itching, high blood pressure

(19) Larch

Larix decidua

For low self-worth

Recommended for those who are lacking self-confidence and feel inferior.

Main symptoms:
- feel insecure and generally expect to fail
- feel useless and impotent; doubt their own abilities; believe that others are cleverer, more beautiful and better
- do not try new things in life because of a conviction they will fail
- anticipate that things will go wrong,

expecting set-backs from whatever action
is taken
- highly self-critical
- fear of examinations, interviews, etc.

Possible physical symptoms:
- alcoholism, impotence, problems or
weakness of the spine, osteoporosis

(20) Mimulus

Mimulus guttatus

For known fears

Recommended for those who are shy and
timid and fear specific things, but tend to
keep it to themselves.

Main symptoms:
- phobias or fears of specific things, such as
hospitals, dentists, syringes, illness, cancer,

heights, flying, crowds, the dark, death, loneliness, animals (dogs, snakes, spiders)…
- easily nervous and intimidated
- avoid certain situations or tasks because of fear; may even fall ill in order to avoid them
- highly sensitive to all kinds of things (noise, smells, cold, bright light)

Possible physical symptoms:
- nervousness, stuttering, blush easily; bladder and kidney problems

(21) Mustard

Sinapis arvensis

For depression

Recommended for those who suffer from depression which comes suddenly and for no apparent reason.

Main symptoms:
- sadness descends like a dark cloud and is all-enveloping
- feel cut off from the rest of the world, desperate and sad, miserable and melancholic
- nothing interests or motivates; a desire to just sit around and do nothing
- there is no logical explanation why this depressive bout strikes; it comes and goes suddenly and there is a sense of profound relief when it has passed

Possible physical symptoms:
- fatigue, weakness, slow movements

(22) Oak

Quercus robur

For endurance

Recommended for those who have overdone it and exhausted themselves.

Main symptoms:
- normally strong and courageous there is now an imminent mental and physical collapse. Can't fight anymore – be it illness or adversity, completely exhausted, but cannot admit it and do not complain about it
- cannot accept help and ignore all signs which indicate the need to rest
- push themselves beyond their limits
- inflexible, stubborn and unrelenting

Possible physical symptoms:
- exhaustion, fatigue, grinding teeth, tension, stiffness and inflexibility of body and mind,

arteriosclerosis, gall-bladder or kidney stones, high blood pressure, high cholesterol

(23) Olive

Olea europaea

For mental and physical exhaustion

Recommended for those who are mentally and physically completely shattered and weak.

Main symptoms:
- weariness and exhaustion, feel worn out
- drained of any energy, washed out, everything is too much of an effort
- constant tiredness – need a lot of sleep
- feel weak and debilitated, daily life is a struggle and joyless

- overworked, the batteries are completely flat, need a lot of rest

Possible physical symptoms:
- weakness and fatigue (e.g. during and after an exhausting illness), weakness of organs such as the heart or thyroid, suffer after-effects of intoxication (drugs, alcohol)

(24) Pine

Pinus sylvestris

For self-blame

Recommended for those who easily feel guilty, constantly apologize and blame themselves.

Main symptoms:
- never content with own efforts, constantly self-critical, even if successful

- apologize all the time for what they are or what they have or have not done, for being ill or tired, etc.
- blame themselves, feel guilty about 'sins' committed and punish themselves
- feel guilty for the faults or mistakes of others
- work very hard and have high expectations of themselves, perfectionists
- feel themselves worthless and inferior

Possible physical symptoms:
- exhaustion, weakness, sexual problems

(25) Red Chestnut

Aesulus carnea

For over-concern

Recommended for those who obsessively worry about others.

Main symptoms:
- constant worry and concern about others, but do not worry about themselves
- over-caring and overprotecting of loved ones, often imagine that something awful has happened to them (e.g. if a child comes home late)
- cannot stop worrying about family, friends or clients
- cannot let go of loved ones
- feel the need to help others

Possible physical symptoms:
- tension, restlessness, insomnia, nervous conditions, heart, circulatory and respiratory problems caused by worry

(26) Rock Rose

Heliathemum nummularium

For terror and panic

Recommended for those who are suffering from acute and extreme fears.

Main symptoms:
- sudden panic, great fear, a feeling of terror (e.g. after accidents, trauma, emergencies, bad news)
- sensation of being paralysed, frayed nerves, unable to think or act rationally
- panic attacks
- a tendency to panic easily, a weak nervous system
- nightmares, sudden anxieties, intoxication by drugs

Possible physical symptoms:
- shock, trembling, palpitations, sweating

(27) Rock Water

Welsh spring water

For inflexibility and self-denial

Recommended for those who are rigid, inflexible and strict with themselves.

Main symptoms:
- strive for perfectionism, need to push themselves to achieve high goals
- strict with themselves, deny themselves pleasure in life, quick to administer self-punishment
- highly disciplined; suppress vital needs, such as sleep, hunger, breaks from work
- follow strict rules in life, such as not drinking alcohol, not eating meat, not smoking, etc.
- rigid opinions and stubborn beliefs

Possible physical symptoms:
- physical rigidity and inflexibility, such as tension, stiffness, rheumatism, arteriosclerosis, gall-bladder or kidney stones

(28) Scleranthus

Scleranthus annuus

For lack of equilibrium and mood swings

Recommended for those who are indecisive, uncertain and moody.

Main-symptoms:
- cannot make up their minds, cannot choose between two options, hesitant
- mood swings, emotional ups-and-downs
- constant changes of opinion

- unable to concentrate, jump from one subject to another
- unreliable, unstable personalities

Possible physical symptoms:
- constant changing symptoms or pains, which may come and go; symptoms of an imbalance, such as vertigo, travel sickness; fluctuating temperatures, changing appetite, bulimia, diarrhoea alternating with constipation

(29) Star of Bethlehem

Ornithogalum umbellatum

For shock

Recommended for those who have experienced a mental or physical shock or trauma.

Main symptoms:
- after-effects from every kind of physical, mental or emotional shock, such as accidents, bad news, disappointments; symptoms can include nightmares, grief, depression, unhappiness, fears, etc. (such a shock can have happened long ago and may have been suppressed and caused all kinds of mental or physical symptoms)
- feel unhappy, but do not want to be comforted

Possible physical symptoms:
- illness after shock; 'incurable' disease, pain, stiffness, arthritis, problems with vision or hearing

(30) Sweet Chestnut

Castanea sativa

For desperation

Recommended for those who are suffering deep anguish and despair.

Main symptoms:
- feel lost, dejected, without any hope
- feel as if the limits of endurance have been reached
- no energy left to fight; on the verge of a mental and physical breakdown
- feel exhausted and worn out, do not think it possible to carry on
- deep depression and despondency
- do not see a solution to their problems, may feel suicidal

Possible physical symptoms:
- physical breakdown

(31) Vervain

Verbena officinalis

For over-enthusiasm

Recommended for those who are fanatical in their beliefs, and end up feeling tense, stressed, worn out and strained.

Main symptoms:
- very convinced about their beliefs and ideas – fanatics, reformers, martyrs, idealists
- overwork in the name of idealism, give their all, push themselves to the brink of a breakdown
- do not listen to other people's advice, but try to convert them
- unable to relax

Possible physical symptoms:
- stress signs such as tension, irritation,

headaches, exhaustion, insomnia, nervousness, restlessness, high blood pressure, colds, stuttering

(32) Vine

Vitis viniferra

For domination

Recommended for those who are very self-confident, powerful, dominating, bossy.

Main symptoms:
- tyrannical, dictatorial
- wilful, pushy and selfish
- lacking sympathy for others
- like to give orders and do not accept contradiction
- like to be powerful, to dominate others, to play power games

- convinced they must be right; inflexible, pedantic and intolerant

Possible physical symptoms:
- pain, tension, stiffness of joints, arterio-sclerosis, high blood pressure, liver problems

(33) Walnut

Juglans regia

For life changes

Recommended for those who struggle with changes in their lives and find it hard to move on.

Main symptoms:
- difficulty in coping with major life changes such as a divorce, moving to a new country, starting a new job, etc.
- have decided to take an important new step in life, but feel hesitant about going ahead

with it; oversensitive to ideas and influences

- feel uneasy about transition, suddenly lack confidence
- have made the transition but cannot adapt to the new situation, cannot move on

Possible physical symptoms:
- complaints and conditions related to a life change such as teething, puberty, pregnancy, menopause; problems of the skin (acne), etc.

(34) Water Violet

Hottonia palustris

For seclusion

Recommended for those who are shy, independent, proud, detached and prefer to be on their own.

Main symptoms:
- problems making contact with other people, even though quite self-confident when alone
- may come across as arrogant, untouchable, remote, unapproachable or disdainful to others
- tendency to feel superior and proud
- try to solve their problems on their own
- rarely weep in front of others
- do not interfere in other people's lives

Possible physical symptoms:
- pain, tension and stiffness, e.g. in back, neck, joints; skin problems

(35) White Chestnut

Aesculus hippocastanum

For mental over-activity

Recommended for those who cannot shut down their mind and have persistent, repetitive and unwanted thoughts.

Main symptoms:
- constant mental arguments and inner conversations, as if a tape is being played over and over again
- persistent worrying; unwanted thoughts and pictures come to mind
- unable to concentrate, disorganized, become depressed
- can't fall asleep or wake up early in the morning

Possible physical symptoms:
- exhaustion, fatigue, tension, headaches, grinding of teeth

(36)
Wild Oat

Bromus ramonus

For uncertainty

Recommended for those who do not know what they want and feel unsure about their purpose in life.

Main symptoms:
- have lots of ideas and plans, but cannot decide what to do
- dissatisfied or desperate, because of feeling uncertain as to what to do next
- have many talents and abilities, but cannot determine their true vocation in life; forever starting something new, such as a new job, a new relationship, etc.
- feel frustrated and unfulfilled in life because of an unsatisfactory situation

(private or professional) e.g. midlife crisis

Possible physical symptoms:
• sexual problems, eating disorders

(37)
Wild Rose

Rosa canina

For resignation and apathy

Recommended for those who lack vitality, have given up on getting any better and suffer from apathy.

Main symptoms:
• lack any joy in life and feel detached from their emotions and feelings
• submit to fate, do not change an unsatisfactory situation (such as illness, an unhappy relationship or unsatisfactory

job) and do not complain about it
- lack ambition and zest, feel dull, monotonous and disinterested
- feel 'floppy', without energy; have a flat voice
- feel hopeless and unmotivated; fatalistic

Possible physical symptoms:
- fatigue, tiredness (from anaemia, chronic disease, weakness of the heart or the thyroid, etc.)

(38) Willow

Salix vitellina

For bitterness and resentment

Recommended for those who are resentful, angry and bitter.

Main symptoms:
- feel negative, resentful and full of self-pity, think they have been treated unfairly
- see only the negative side of things
- blame others for their misfortune
- envy others for their fortune, health, etc.
- feel a victim of circumstance
- full of suppressed anger, but do not explode (like a smouldering volcano)
- constantly demand attention and help but not prepared to give to others

Possible physical symptoms:
- problems with the skin, gall-bladder and liver; rheumatism

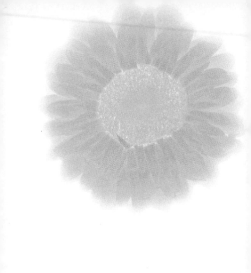

PART
THREE

EMOTIONAL COMPLAINTS
FROM A TO Z

Edward Bach listed his remedies under seven different headings. He differentiated between remedies for treating fear (page 102), uncertainty (page 135), insufficient interest in present circumstances (page 109), loneliness (page 112), oversensitivity to influences and ideas (page 120), despondency and despair (page 98), and for people who are over-caring and demanding (page 118).

This chapter contains these and many more emotional complaints, all listed in alphabetical order.

To find the right remedy for your condition, look under the appropriate heading and compare the description of each remedy with the symptoms of your complaint. Choose the Bach Remedies associated with the symptoms which most closely correspond to your condition. If several remedies seem applicable, cross-check them with the profiles of each remedy in the chapter The Complete Remedies from A to Z, starting on page 34.

For the limitations of self-treatment refer to page 188 (When should you seek professional help?). Where indicated with an asterisk (*) it is highly recommended that you seek professional advice.

ABSENT-MINDEDNESS

- If you spend your time day-dreaming, lack concentration, do not pay attention, repeat the same mistakes and tend to lose things easily or seek to escape from reality into the future, *Clematis* is the right choice.
- If you dwell on the past, *Honeysuckle* is better.
- If persistent repetitive thoughts are the reason for absent-mindedness, *White Chestnut* is extremely effective.
- Do you repeat the same mistakes over and over again? Do you feel easily confused, scatty and unable to concentrate? In this case take *Chestnut Bud*.

ACCEPTANCE, lack of

See page 133 – Tolerance, lack of

AGGRESSION, ANGER, RAGE

- *Holly* is the most important remedy for any kind of negative and destructive emotion, such as anger, hatred, rage, jealousy, suspicion, etc. Even violence and choleric behaviour can be eased with this Bach Remedy.
- *Willow* is extremely useful for those who are resentful and bitter.
- If you are irritable and impatient because others are much slower than yourself, try *Impatiens*.
- If you are critical and intolerant of other people or of other people's habits, consider *Beech*.
- If you get angry when others do not follow your orders or even contradict you, *Vine* is recommended.
- Do you feel angry because other people have different ideals, beliefs or opinions? Then *Vervain* can be very effective.

AMBITION, lacking

- For those who lack self-confidence and doubt very much that they will be successful, *Larch* is very reliable.
- If you lack vitality, feel dull and disinterested or quite fatalistic, take *Wild Rose*.
- For those who are absent-minded, day-dreamers, or who simply try to escape reality and spend hours in front of computer games or the TV, *Clematis* is helpful.

AMBITIOUS, too

- If you are over-enthusiastic and fanatical in your beliefs and you want everyone to feel the same, consider *Vervain*.
- *Rock Water* is a helpful remedy in cases where you strive for too much perfection and push yourself to achieve

high goals. You tend to be highly
disciplined.

- If you like to be powerful and to
  dominate others, and you push or
  manipulate people for your own benefit,
  take *Vine*.
- If you are ambitious and push yourself
  until you are utterly exhausted, then *Oak*
  may be the remedy.
- If it is all-important for you to be
  accepted and climb up the social ladder,
  Heather is the appropriate remedy.

ANGER

See page 87 – Aggression

ANXIETY

See page 102 – Fearfulness

APATHY

See page 111 – Lethargy

ARROGANCE

- You may seem arrogant to others, because you are independent and self-confident. But if you are rather shy and prefer to be on your own, take *Water Violet*.
- If you think you know what is best for other people, try *Vine*.
- If intolerance is the reason for behaving in an arrogant manner, *Beech* is the best remedy.
- If you seem arrogant but this is actually due to a feeling of deep insecurity, *Larch* can give you more self-confidence.

ATTENTION SEEKING

- If you constantly need people around you to talk about yourself and your problems, *Heather* is the right remedy.
- If you often seek out the attention of your family, partner or friends, if you worry about them, cannot let go of them and are deeply hurt if they seem to neglect you, take *Chicory*.

BAD TEMPERED

See page 92 – Choleric

BITTERNESS, RESENTFULNESS

- If you feel bitter and resentful, *Willow* is helpful

CHOLERIC, BAD TEMPERED

- If you easily explode and suffer from outbursts of anger, *Holly* is the best remedy.
- If you fear you are losing control, take *Cherry Plum*.

CONCENTRATION, lack of

- When mistakes are repeated over and over again and you do not learn from experience, take *Chestnut Bud*.
- If you have persistent thoughts, internal arguments and conversations, *Wild Chestnut* is the best remedy to help to settle and quieten down your mind.
- If you are day-dreaming and escaping from reality into the future, *Clematis* is recommended.

- If you dwell more in the past *Honeysuckle* will be better.

- If impatience and restlessness prevent you from concentrating, consider *Impatiens*.

- If you have so many ideas and plans that you cannot concentrate on one, try *Wild Oat*.

- Should you get easily distracted or keep jumping from one subject to another and are quite moody, *Scleranthus* helps.

CONTROL, losing*

- When you feel emotionally extremely blocked and frightened of losing control, take *Cherry Plum*. *Rescue Remedy* also contains Cherry Plum and can be used instead.

COURAGE, lack of

- Take either *Mimulus* for specific fears or *Aspen* for general apprehension and anxiety.
- Use *Centaury* if you are weak-willed and easily exploited.
- If you lack self-confidence, *Larch* is highly recommended.
- If a shocking event or experience is the reason for your lack of courage, then *Star of Bethlehem* is a wonderful help.
- If you try to avoid confrontation, because you cannot tolerate conflict and arguments, the best remedy is *Agrimony*.
- If you feel easily discouraged see page 99 – Discouragement.

DEMANDING

See page 118 – Over-caring

DEPENDENCY

- For being unable to say 'no', being easily influenced, even bullied by others *Centaury* is recommended.
- If you do not trust your own judgment and constantly have to ask other people for advice, take *Cerato*.
- Those who cannot be on their own and constantly need to talk about themselves, should try *Heather*.
- If you need another's protection because you are afraid of other people or certain situations, you will benefit from *Mimulus*.
- If you are caring of others, but also need their appreciation and feel easily hurt or unloved if you do not get it, *Chicory* will free you of this dependency.

DEPRESSION*

- The main Bach Remedy for depression is *Mustard*. You feel as if sadness descends upon you like a dark cloud. This comes and goes for no apparent reason.

- *Gentian* helps when you know why you are depressed. Difficulties, set-backs and failures trigger the depression.
- Do you also feel bitter and resentful? In this case *Willow* will be useful.
- If there is also a lot of anger and aggression, *Holly* is more appropriate.
- Depression caused by shock responds well to *Star of Bethlehem*.
- If you have given up all hope and feel over-tired and depressed, *Gorse* can be helpful.
- If you have submitted to your fate, feel apathetic and fatalistic, consider *Wild Rose*.
- If you feel physically and mentally exhausted, try *Olive*.
- If you suddenly feel overwhelmed by responsibilities and tasks, *Elm* is a reliable remedy.
- *Crab Apple* is helpful in cases where you cannot accept yourself and are depressed

because you feel contaminated, unclean or dirty.

- If you feel guilty and depressed, try *Pine*.
- If anxiety is the reason for your depressive mood, *Aspen* is a reliable remedy.
- If you are brooding and dwelling in the past, you should think about *Honeysuckle*.
- If you do not feel loved, *Chicory* will bring relief.
- *Heather* helps if you feel abandoned and rejected.
- Those who experience deep anguish and despair should take *Sweet Chestnut*.
- Do you lack self-confidence and feel constantly inferior? In this case *Larch* will help.

DESPAIR

See page 98 – Despondency

DESPONDENCY* and DESPAIR*

- For a lack of self-confidence, feelings of insecurity and expectations of failure, consider taking *Larch*. It is the main remedy for low self-worth.

- If you feel easily guilty and often blame yourself, *Pine* is preferable.

- If you are suddenly overburdened and exhausted and you do not know how to cope anymore, take *Elm*.

- For deep despair, feeling you have reached the limits of your endurance, *Sweet Chestnut* is extremely helpful.

- For the after-effects of all kinds of physical, mental or emotional shock (such as bad news, accidents or disappointments), consider *Star of Bethlehem*.

- Should you feel bitter, resentful and let down by life, *Willow* will be the best.

- If you suffer from exhaustion, despondency and despair because you constantly fight against obstacles, try *Oak*.
- Those who feel unclean, dirty and infected, or feel desperate to wash or tidy up, should consider *Crab Apple*. It is the cleanser of the Bach Remedies.

DISAPPOINTMENT

See below – Discouragement

DISCOURAGEMENT, DISAPPOINTMENT, DOUBT

- If things have not worked out as you wanted and you are sceptical and doubtful, the remedy most likely to help is *Gentian*.
- If you are disappointed because your family or friends neglect you, consider *Chicory*.
- Take *Elm* if you feel suddenly overwhelmed

by some task or test.
* Should you also feel bitter and resentful, take *Willow*.

DISGUST

* Those who feel unclean, 'dirty' or full of self-disgust, who have an excessive need to wash, to clean and to tidy up, will benefit from *Crab Apple*.
* For disgust and intolerance consider *Beech*.

DISTRACTION

* If you feel easily confused, scatty and absent-minded, repeat the same mistakes and have a tendency to lose things, *Chestnut Bud* is the right choice.
* If you feel there are so many possibilities and options you cannot make up your mind which one to follow, *Wild Oat* is the best remedy to take.

- For those who are unable to concentrate, who keep jumping from one subject to another or are moody, *Scleranthus* is very effective.

DOMINATION

- If you try to dominate other people and push them to do what you want, try *Vine*.
- If you are over-enthusiastic or fanatical in your beliefs, ideas and plans and you push others to act the way you do, *Vervain* is the better choice.
- If you try to manipulate and dominate your family or friends, take *Chicory*.

DOUBT

See page 99 – Discouragement

ENVY

- If you lack self-confidence, *Larch* is helpful.
- Take *Holly* if you feel powerful negative emotions such as anger, rage, etc.
- If you also feel bitter and resentful, *Willow* is recommended.

EXPLOITATION

- If you feel easily exploited by your family or friends, *Chicory* is the right remedy.
- If other people easily exploit you because you are weak willed, *Centaury* is the better choice.

FEARFULNESS*, ANXIETY*

- If you suffer from acute panic attacks, extreme fears and terror, e.g. after an accident, take *Rock Rose*.

- For the fear of losing control, of going mad or having a nervous breakdown when under extreme pressure, *Cherry Plum* will bring relief.

- If you experience fear of specific things, such as illness, death, flying, etc., you may benefit from *Mimulus* as it is the main Bach Remedy for phobias.

- For anxiety about unknown things, a vague feeling of fear, apprehension and panic, take *Aspen*.

- In cases where you worry too much about people close to you (such as family, friends or clients), *Red Chestnut* is very effective.

FORGETFULNESS

- For those who have difficulty with studying and tend to make the same mistakes over and over again, *Chestnut Bud* is best.

- If you tend to suppress or forget worrying thoughts and problems, *Agrimony* helps.
- If a trauma has caused some kind of amnesia, try *Star of Bethlehem*.
- If you don't listen or pay attention because you are too absorbed with your own problems, consider *Heather*.
- If you are dreamy and inattentive *Clematis* or *Red Chestnut* is helpful.
- If you cannot concentrate, see page xx – Concentration, lack of.

GRIEF, LOVESICKNESS

- The main remedy for the shock of losing someone or something you greatly value is *Star of Bethlehem*.
- If you hide your true feelings and put on a brave face, take *Agrimony*.
- If repetitive thoughts torment you and prevent you from sleeping, *White*

Chestnut is useful.

- If you dwell on past memories, *Red Chestnut* will be what you need.
- If you feel possessive and you cannot let go, try *Chicory*.
- For deep despair, *Sweet Chestnut* is an effective remedy.
- For depression and pessimism after grief, *Gentian* is recommended.
- If you feel jealousy or hate, take *Holly*.
- If your self-confidence is in tatters, *Larch* is helpful.
- For bitterness, *Willow* is the appropriate choice.
- Do you find that you prefer to be alone? If so, consider *Water Violet*.

GUILT COMPLEX

- For those who feel easily guilty, constantly apologize and blame themselves, *Pine* is appropriate.

HOMESICKNESS

- If you feel homesick, take *Honeysuckle*.

HOPELESSNESS

- If set-backs and failures are the reason for feeling depressed, discouraged and losing hope, take *Gentian*.
- If you feel defeated and deeply depressed, consider *Gorse*, the main remedy for hopelessness.
- If depression descends like a dark cloud and you feel deeply sad and cut off from the world, *Mustard* will help.
- If you feel deep despair and as if you have reached the limits of your endurance, *Sweet Chestnut* is best.
- Fatalism, resignation, apathy and a lack of vitality respond well to *Wild Rose*.

HUMILIATION

- For shock *Star of Bethlehem* or *Rescue Remedy* bring relief.
- Those who are self-obsessed and vain tend to suffer most from humiliation. *Heather* will help in these cases.

INDECIVENESS

- When you are indecisive and you cannot make up your mind which of two different options to choose, *Scleranthus* will be the right remedy.
- If you feel torn and uncertain because you have many ideas and options and you cannot determine what to do in life, *Wild Oat* will help, especially if you feel dissatisfied.

INDIFFERENCE

See page 109 – Interest in the present, lack of

INFERIORITY COMPLEX

See page 124 – Self-confidence, lack of

INFLEXIBILITY

- For those who are rigid, inflexible and strict with themselves, *Rock Water* is recommended.
- If you are stubborn, inflexible and unrelenting and push yourself beyond your limits, *Oak* will be the better choice.
- For those who tend to dominate others and cannot accept or tolerate other opinions, *Vine* is the right remedy.
- Those who are fanatical in their beliefs and cannot tolerate other people's points of view benefit from Vervain.

INTEREST IN THE PRESENT, lack of; INDIFFERENCE

- For dreaminess, drowsiness and fantasizing about the future or escaping from reality by watching TV, playing computer games, taking drugs, etc., *Clematis* is extremely effective.

- If you dwell on the past, are nostalgic or even homesick, *Honeysuckle* is the best remedy.

- If you have submitted to your fate, feel fatalistic and lacking in vitality, *Wild Rose* will help.

- If you feel mentally and physically completely exhausted and overworked, then take *Olive*, especially if daily life has become a struggle.

- For mental over-activity and constant inner conversations and dialogue which prevent you from concentrating on life in the present, *White Chestnut* is helpful.

- If you do not pay attention to the lessons of life and seem to repeat the same mistakes over and over again, consider *Chestnut Bud*.
- Should you suffer from depression which suddenly comes and descends like a dark cloud, *Mustard* will be best. Nothing can interest or motivate you at such times.

JEALOUSY

- The main Bach Remedy for this emotional state is *Holly*.
- If you cannot let go of someone beloved, take *Chicory*.
- For jealousy mixed with bitterness, *Willow* can bring good results.

KEEP SMILING

- For those who try to hide their worries and anxieties behind humour and a brave face, *Agrimony* will be a soothing remedy.

LET GO, cannot

- If you are under a lot of strain and you fear losing control, *Cherry Plum* is best.
- If you cannot let go of a beloved person or possession *Chicory* or *Red Chestnut* will be helpful.
- If you cannot let go of certain thoughts, which constantly come back to haunt you, *White Chestnut* is preferable.

LETHARGY and APATHY

- For those who lack vitality, have given up any hope of recovery and suffer from resignation or apathy, *Wild Rose* is the main remedy.
- If you also feel sad and depressed, try *Mustard*.
- For lethargy caused by mental and/or physical exhaustion, you should take *Olive*.

- If you feel 'floppy' and lethargic in the morning but better throughout the day, *Hornbeam* is reliable.

LONELINESS

- For those who try to solve their problems on their own and prefer to be alone, *Water Violet* will help them to become less isolated and reserved.

- If you are rather irritable and impatient with the slowness of others and therefore prefer to be on your own, *Impatiens* is the right remedy.

- If you cannot be on your own and constantly seek companionship because you have to talk to someone about your problems, *Heather* will help you to become less self-obsessed.

LOVESICKNESS

See page 104 – Grief

MANIPULATION

- If you are easily manipulated because you cannot say 'no', *Centaury* should be considered.
- If you do not trust your own opinions and you constantly have to ask others for advice, *Cerato* is the better choice.
- For a general lack of self-confidence, *Larch* should be taken.
- Consider *Walnut* if you are in a stage of transition. At such times you may feel vulnerable and find that you are easily manipulated.
- If you tend to manipulate your family, partner or friends, simply because you think it is best for them, *Chicory* is a good choice.

- For manipulative behaviour arising from fanatical zeal, consider *Vervain*.
- Those who manipulate and dominate others and cannot accept contradiction will benefit from *Vine*.

MOOD SWINGS

- If you cannot decide between two options, if you are indecisive, and suffer from mood swings and emotional ups-and-downs, *Scleranthus* is the appropriate remedy.
- If you do not know what you want because there are so many possibilities, options, ideas and plans to choose from, *Wild Oat* is the better choice.
- If you do not trust your own judgement and always have to ask others for advice, *Cerato* will help.

NERVOUS BREAKDOWN*

- If you are emotionally extremely blocked and you fear that you are losing control, *Cherry Plum* will calm you down. As it is one of the *Rescue Remedy* ingredients you can take that instead.

- If shock led to a nervous breakdown, *Star of Bethlehem* is best. As above, you can take *Rescue Remedy* instead.

- For acute exhaustion, stress and feeling overwhelmed by responsibilities, *Elm* is advisable.

- For those who have overdone it and have become exhausted over a long period by pushing themselves beyond their limits, or those who have refused to be helped and ignored all danger signs, *Oak* is helpful.

- If you suffer deep anguish and despair and you do not think you can carry on, *Sweet Chestnut* will help.

NERVOUSNESS*

- If you are nervous and fearful, *Mimulus* can bring fast relief.
- Are you impatient and always in a hurry? If so take *Impatiens*.
- A lack of self-confidence often responds well to *Larch*.
- Take *Elm* if you are nervous and exhausted.
- For nervousness caused by fears and anxieties which you keep hidden behind a mask of humour and jolliness, *Agrimony* is an effective remedy.
- If you worry so much about other people that it makes you nervous, *Red Chestnut* will help.
- If you are nervous about other people or crowds, *Water Violet* is recommended.

NIGHTMARES

- *Rock Rose* is commonly used for acute and extreme fear, such as when you wake from a nightmare. It is part of the *Rescue Remedy*, so you could take that instead.
- If you have problems getting back to sleep because you feel anxious and panicky, you need *Aspen*.
- Nightmares caused by some shocking event respond well to *Star of Bethlehem*.
- Take *Aspen* for anxiety, and *Mimulus* for fear and to help reduce scary nightmares and the fear of having them.
- Are the nightmares caused by some feeling of guilt? If so, *Pine* is preferable.

OVERACTIVE MIND

- Those who cannot settle their mind and have persistent, repetitive and unwanted thoughts benefit most from *White Chestnut*.

- If you think much faster than others and you easily get impatient and annoyed, take *Impatiens*.
- If you constantly dwell on the past, try *Honeysuckle*.

OVER-CARING and DEMANDING

- If you are caring of others, but also need their appreciation and feel easily hurt or unloved if you do not get it, or if you tend to be demanding and manipulative, *Chicory* will be best.
- For fanatical over-caring people, reformers and idealists who overwork and exhaust themselves, *Vervain* is very good.
- If you like to give orders or try to dominate others because you are convinced you know what is best for them, try *Vine*.

- If you constantly notice other people's mistakes and tend to be critical and intolerant, *Beech* is probably the right remedy for you.
- Should you expect too much of yourself and be rather too hard on yourself, you will need *Rock Water*.

OVERSENSITIVITY

- If you are lacking self-confidence and you are oversensitive to criticism, you should consider *Larch*.
- If you cannot bear quarrels and disputes, you will respond well to *Agrimony*.
- *Mimulus* helps if you are rather shy, timid and oversensitive to noise.
- If you are oversensitive to dirt, infections, pollution, smells or untidiness, take *Crab Apple*.

OVERSENSITIVENESS
to influences and ideas

- If you avoid and reject anything which might disturb your peace and harmony, *Agrimony* will help to ease your anxiety and worries, especially if you have a tendency to hide your true feelings behind a mask of cheerfulness.

- For those who are easily influenced by others because they lack self-confidence and cannot say 'no', *Centaury* works extremely well. It helps them to become more assertive.

- If you experience a change in your life (physically or emotionally) and you feel uneasy about the transition, you should try *Walnut*. It will help you to adapt to new situations.

- If you suffer from negative emotional states, such as anger, envy, jealousy, hatred, suspicion, etc., *Holly* will bring relief.

PANIC*

- The first remedy you should consider for acute and extreme fears, feelings of terror and panic attacks is *Rock Rose*. If some shocking event or trauma is the reason for your panic, add *Star of Bethlehem*. If you feel you are losing control, *Cherry Plum* is the best. All of these three Bach Remedies are part of the *Rescue Remedy*, which can be used instead.

- If stress causes panic, *Elm* will be helpful.

- If you are anxious and frequently feel panicky for no apparent reason, *Aspen* will give you strength.

- Are you worrying and panicky about those you love? *Red Chestnut* can be very effective.

PESSIMISM

- If it is caused by disappointments, failure and set-backs, *Gentian* is very useful.
- If it is caused by bitterness, *Willow* will be better.
- Have you given up hope? If so, *Gorse* is more appropriate.
- *Elm* should be considered if stress and acute exhaustion are the cause.
- If you feel very pessimistic in the morning but your mood improves during the day, try *Hornbeam*.

POSSESSIVENESS

- For those who are over-preoccupied with their loved ones' well-being, are demanding, interfering and manipulative, *Chicory* is the most suitable remedy.

RAGE

See page 87 – Aggression

RESENTFUL

See page 91 – Bitterness

RESIGNATION

- The best remedy is *Wild Rose*.
- If you also feel there is no hope any more, add *Gorse*.

RESTLESSNESS

- If you feel impatient and irritable, *Impatiens* will be the right choice.
- If you hide your fears, worries and restlessness behind humour and a brave face, *Agrimony* is the better remedy.
- If you do not trust your own judgement and you constantly ask others for advice,

Cerato will give you more confidence.

- Restlessness of the mind, which prevents you from sleeping or calming down, responds well to *White Chestnut*.
- If guilt makes you feel restless, consider *Pine*.
- If you worry too much about others, then *Red Chestnut* is recommended.
- If fears makes you restless, *Mimulus* is helpful.
- For those who need constant attention and get very restless when alone, *Heather* is useful.

SELF-CONFIDENCE, lack of; INFERIORITY COMPLEX

- The main remedy to boost your self-confidence is *Larch*.
- If you have to ask constantly for advice, *Cerato* is very helpful too.
- If you are weak willed, add *Centaury*.

SELFISHNESS

- For those who are possessive of their loved ones, are constantly criticizing them and are self-preoccupied, *Chicory* is very useful.
- If you are obsessed with yourself and need to be the centre of attention, *Heather* is the best remedy.
- If you are wilful, pushy or dictatorial, like to dominate others and tend to be very self-righteous, *Vine* is more appropriate.
- *Vervain* should be considered for those who are fanatical in their beliefs and do not listen to other people's advice. They also have a tendency to be self-righteous.

SELF-PITY

- Those who feel sorry for themselves often benefit from *Chicory*.
- If you feel easily humiliated, consider *Heather*.

SHOCK, TRAUMA*

- For those who have experienced some form of shock and trauma (even if it was a long time ago), *Star of Bethlehem* is most helpful.
- For acute shock and trauma *Rescue Remedy* is the better choice, as it also contains remedies for panic, loss of control and fainting.

SHOWING OFF

- If you feel inferior and need to prove your worth to others, *Larch* will boost your confidence.
- In cases where you want to make yourself seem more interesting and you want to impress others, take *Heather*. It is often helpful to combine the two remedies.

STAMINA, lack of

- If you give up because you feel discouraged, *Gentian* should be considered first.

- If you lack stamina because you cannot decide between two options, take *Scleranthus*. Should you have many ideas and plans but cannot make up your mind what to do and what to pursue, *Wild Oat* is the better choice.

- If you lack the energy to go on, *Olive* – the remedy for exhaustion – should be taken.

- Consider *Wild Rose* if you have given up and submitted to your fate. You feel resignation, apathy and a lack of vitality.

- You have fought long and hard, but you cannot go on any more and you are on the brink of giving up. In this case *Oak* is a good choice.

- If you have given up all hope and deep

inside you feel very pessimistic and
beyond help, *Gorse* is very useful.

STRESS

- If you feel acutely stressed, weak and
  exhausted by overwhelming
  responsibilities, *Elm* is recommended.
- If you feel extremely stressed and
  uptight, as if you are losing control or
  sitting on a time bomb which could
  explode at any minute, *Cherry Plum* is
  best.
- For those who hide their tensions,
  problems and anxieties behind a brave
  face, *Agrimony* is extremely effective.
- If you get easily stressed because you are
  irritable and impatient, take *Impatiens*.
- If you are over-enthusiastic in your
  beliefs and you end up feeling tense,
  stressed, worn out and strained, consider
  Vervain.

- If you push yourself beyond your limits, *Oak* is recommended.
- If fears are causing stress, *Mimulus* is helpful.

SUBMISSIVENESS

- For those who are weak willed, easily exploited or imposed upon, *Centaury* will be best.

SUICIDAL*

- For this acute feeling *Rescue Remedy* can help. But you should also get professional advice (e.g. GP or via a telephone helpline).
- If you feel emotionally extremely blocked and fear you are losing control, *Cherry Plum* is the best remedy.
- If you are in deep despair, take *Sweet Chestnut*.

- For depression which descends like a dark cloud, give *Mustard*.
- If you have given up all hope, *Gorse* is preferable.
- Do you hide your worries and problems behind a brave face and tell the world you are all right? In this case *Agrimony* will help.
- If you avoid problems by withdrawing into a world of your own and you even welcome the prospect of death, *Clematis* is a good choice.

SULKINESS

- If you sulk because you do not get what you want from others, or if you do not get enough gratitude, attention or sympathy, try *Chicory*.
- If you feel bitter and resentful because you think you have been treated unfairly, *Willow* is preferable.

SUPERSTITIOUSNESS

- For a general vague feeling of fear or danger, fear of ghosts or places or situations, *Aspen* is the best remedy.

SUPPRESSION

- If you hide worries and anxieties behind humour and a brave face, *Agrimony* is helpful.

TIREDNESS

- Those who suffer from mental exhaustion, feel tired, 'floppy' and heavy, or wearied by the same job or the same situation, can benefit from *Hornbeam*.
- If you are tired because you feel overburdened by tasks and responsibilities, the most important remedy is *Elm*.
- If you feel physically and mentally

exhausted, tired and weak, take *Olive*.

- You have pushed yourself beyond your limits and ignored all signs telling you to rest. You know you have overdone it, but you do not want to be helped. If so, *Oak* is recommended.

- For those who are over-enthusiastic about their ideas and beliefs and end up feeling worn out, stressed and tired, *Vervain* is helpful.

- If you lack joy and energy, feel 'floppy', dull or disinterested and detached from your emotions, *Wild Rose* is excellent.

- Do you feel tired because you cannot say 'no' to others and therefore give them too much of your energy and time? In this case take *Centaury*.

- If you feel tired because you worry and care obsessively for others, *Red Chestnut* is best.

- If you believe that you have not done well, or if you constantly push and criticize yourself or apologize to others, *Pine* will bring you some peace of mind.

- Are you avoiding reality, day-dreaming and sleepy? Do you seem absent-minded? In this case *Clematis* is beneficial.

- For tiredness caused by an overactive mind which prevents sleep and relaxation, *Wild Chestnut* should be used.

- If you have given up hope and feel defeated and too tired and depressed to change things for the better, take *Gorse*.

- For tiredness and depression *Mustard* is recommended.

TOLERANCE and ACCEPTANCE, lack of

- The main remedy for intolerance is *Beech*. You can mix it with one of the remedies listed in the rest of this section.

- If you cannot accept or tolerate the opinions of other people, take *Vine*.

- If you cannot accept yourself or constantly criticize yourself, try *Larch*. If you also push or punish yourself, and deny yourself any pleasure in life, *Rock Water* is preferable.
- If you cannot accept or tolerate the situation you are in, and therefore become bitter and resentful, consider *Willow*.
- If you cannot tolerate people who are slower than you, *Impatiens* is best.
- Do you find that you tend to expect other people to share your beliefs/opinions and resent them if they disagree? In this case take *Vervain*.

TRAUMA

See page 126 – Shock

UNCERTAINTY

- *Cerato* can help in cases where you do not trust your own opinion and constantly ask for advice.

- When you are indecisive and cannot make up your mind which of two different options to choose, *Scleranthus* will be the right remedy.

- If you feel torn and uncertain because you have many ideas and options and you cannot determine what to do in life, *Wild Oat* will help, especially if you feel dissatisfied.

- Scepticism, pessimism and discouragement caused by disappointment and frustration are symptoms which respond well to *Gentian*.

- If you have given up hope already and doubt there is anything which will make a difference to your situation, try *Gorse*.

- If you believe that you cannot manage to get through the day, but once you get going you improve, take *Hornbeam*.

UNHAPPINESS

- *Gentian* is an important remedy if you feel disappointed and discouraged.
- If you have no real reason for your unhappiness *Mustard* will help with this kind of mild depression.
- If you are unhappy because you have not found your real purpose in life, try *Wild Oat*.
- If you lack self-confidence and you are unhappy about your weaknesses, consider *Larch*.
- If you are unhappy because you feel guilty about something, *Pine* is recommended.
- If you feel unhappy because you do not get enough attention and love, *Chicory* is helpful.

VANITY

- Those who tend to be obsessed with themselves should take *Heather*.

WORRY

- If you worry obsessively about others in your care, *Red Chestnut* will bring relief.
- If you over-worry about the behaviour of family members, partner or friends (or that they might leave you) *Chicory* is best.
- If you are worried about certain specific things, add *Mimulus*.
- Are you worried that others take advantage of you? In this case take *Heather*.
- For those who worry about being infected, contaminated, 'dirty' or ill, *Crab Apple* is a good remedy.
- If you feel worried but hide it behind humour and a brave face, *Agrimony* will ease hidden anxieties.

PART
FOUR

PHYSICAL COMPLAINTS
FROM A TO Z

Throughout the history of medicine, reference has been made to the connection between mind and body. During the last 100 years we have lost sight of this holistic perspective, but have recently begun to rediscover the interdependence between emotional and physical well-being. This is precisely the premise upon which Bach Remedies are based. Many illnesses in the West are no longer caused by malnutrition or unhygienic conditions, but by emotional problems. Bullying, deprivation of love, anger, lack of self-confidence, anxieties, ambition, humiliation and so on can cause stress. Stress weakens our immune system and causes illness. But illness can also effect our state of mind. It can make us aggressive, irritable or withdrawn. Bach Remedies can help here too.

Bach Remedies can be used *in addition* to medical or complementary treatment for your physical complaints. To treat physical complaints, first try to find those remedies which fit your emotional state, either with the help of the questionnaire or the chapter Emotional Complaints from A to Z starting on page 84.

In this chapter you will find a range of physical complaints for which Bach Remedies are known to be helpful. Compare them with the remedies you chose for yourself in the first instance. Bear in mind that you may have suppressed some emotional trauma or difficult feelings. This can result in a situation where you do not feel the emotional problem but develop a physical condition instead.

Finally you can cross-check the remedies in the chapter The Complete Remedies from A to Z, starting on page 34. For the limitations of self-treatment refer to page 188 (When should you seek professional help?). Where indicated with an asterisk (*) it is highly recommended that you seek professional advice.

> It is important when choosing which remedy to take for a physical complaint that you ask yourself how you are feeling emotionally.

A

ACCIDENTS* and BURNS*

- For all accidents and mild burns take *Rescue Remedy*. You can also apply it externally (see page 14 – Rescue Remedy).

ACNE

- The most important remedy for this condition is *Crab Apple*. *Larch* is helpful if acne undermines your self-confidence. *Walnut* should be used for acne during puberty or the menopause. If it reoccurs periodically, *Chestnut Bud* can be beneficial. All Bach Remedies can also be used externally (see page 182, The Way to Take Bach Remedies).

ALCOHOL

See page 149 – Drugs

ANOREXIA

See page 151 – Eating Disorders

ALLERGIES*

• Take *Beech* for intolerance to allergens (such as food, animal hair, etc.). Take *Walnut* for sensitivity to external influences (such as pollen, etc.) and *Crab Apple* to detox.

BIRTH

See page 164 – Pregnancy

BLOATEDNESS

See page 147 – Digestive Problems

BLOOD PRESSURE, irregular*/DIZZINESS*

- For acute conditions take *Rescue Remedy*.
- If you suffer from low blood pressure, with symptoms such as tiredness, paleness, weakness or dizziness, consider *Clematis*, *Centaury* (weak willed), *Elm* (acute exhaustion), *Olive* (weakness), *Hornbeam* (tiredness) or *Wild Rose* (lack of vitality).
- For high blood pressure with symptoms such as vertigo, headaches or a flushed face, consider *Cherry Plum*. Take *Aspen* if you feel anxious, *Impatiens* if irritable and impatient, *Holly* for anger problems, *Vervain* for over-activity, *Vine* if you tend to dominate others, *Willow* for boiling resentment and *Oak* if you are pushing yourself beyond your limits.
- If your blood pressure goes up and down and you experience mood swings, *Scleranthus* can be helpful.

BULIMIA

See page 151 – Eating Disorders

BURNS

See page 143 – Accidents

COLDS/IMMUNE SYSTEM, weak*

- If you feel mentally or physically exhausted *Olive* is recommended. Take *Crab Apple* too – it cleanses the system. *Walnut* strengthens your system in the face of external influences (such as a flu epidemic) and *Clematis* or *Wild Rose* strengthen your vitality. All the above mentioned remedies can be taken as a preventative. For sudden exhaustion take *Elm*. If you feel aggressive, use *Holly*. If you want love and attention, *Chicory* is helpful. Anger and bitterness can be dealt with by taking *Willow*. If you withdraw and you want to be alone, *Water Violet* is helpful. If your cold is lingering and you get frustrated or desperate, take *Gentian*.

CONSTIPATION

See below – Digestive Problems

DIARRHOEA

See below – Digestive Problems

DIGESTIVE PROBLEMS*, such as CONSTIPATION, DIARRHOEA, BLOATEDNESS

• If you suffer from diarrhoea consider remedies for weakness, such as *Olive*,

Elm, Wild Rose, Clematis. Often fears and anxieties cause loose stools. Here *Aspen*, *Mimulus* and *Rock Rose* as well as *Larch* to boost your confidence, are helpful. If diarrhoea alternates with constipation *Scleranthus* is recommended. Take *Crab Apple* as it helps to detox. *Holly* may be useful for all extreme (violent) conditions.

- For constipation (if you have an emotional difficulty about letting go) consider *Cherry Plum*. If you feel disgusted by your own bowel movements or by unclean toilets (e.g. 'travel constipation') *Crab Apple* helps. It is also a good detox remedy. If you have problems letting go of loved ones and you tend to be possessive or greedy, *Chicory* can help.

- Bloatedness can be related to anger and arrogance. Remedies such as *Holly* (anger), *Willow* (resentment) and *Beech* (food-intolerance), *Vine* (dominance) *Water Violet* (seclusion) or *Heather* (self-absorption) can be taken. But a weak digestion can also cause wind and bloatedness and may be helped by remedies such as *Olive*, *Clematis* and *Wild Rose*. Fast and rushed eating habits can cause indigestion and wind. In this case take *Impatiens*.

- For recurring digestive problems consider *Chestnut Bud* or *Gentian*.

DIZZINESS

See page 145 – Blood Pressure, irregular

DRUGS/ALCOHOL
abuse*, detox*, after-effects*

- If you suppress your problems and anxieties and take alcohol or drugs to dull your inner pain, *Agrimony* is helpful. If you tend to try to escape from reality, consider *Clematis*. A lack of self-confidence can be treated with *Larch*. If you are easily influenced by others, *Centaury* or *Cerato* may be helpful. Take *Star of Bethlehem* if you have experienced something shocking you cannot cope with.

- Take *Crab Apple* for detox. It can also help with the side-effects of drugs (such as a hangover).
- After-effects and withdrawal symptoms: for anxiety use *Aspen*, for sudden panic and terror *Rock Rose*, for fears *Mimulus*, for mental fatigue and hangovers *Hornbeam*. Nervousness and irritability respond to *Impatiens*. If you fear you are losing control take *Cherry Plum*. For extreme exhaustion and fatigue take *Olive*. For obsessive repetitive thoughts *White Chestnut* can help.

EATING DISORDERS*, such as ANOREXIA, BULIMIA

- Eating disorders often accompany, or are triggered by, emotional problems. If you feel unloved and do not get enough care or attention, consider *Chicory*. If an emotional shock triggered the problem, take *Star of Bethlehem*. For fears (e.g. of becoming too fat) *Mimulus* is useful. Take *Agrimony* if you hide your worries and anxieties behind a brave face. For anger and resentment use *Willow*. Other negative emotions like anger, hate, jealousy or envy respond well to *Holly*. If you fear losing control (compulsive/obsessive disorders), take *Cherry Plum*. Take *Crab Apple* for self-disgust. If you feel worthless and inferior *Pine* and *Larch* help. For repetitive obsessive thoughts *White Chestnut* is recommended. *Olive* is useful if you feel weak and exhausted. Do you want to escape from reality? If so, *Clematis* can help. *Scleranthus*, the remedy for imbalance, helps in cases of an erratic appetite or even bulimia. If you feel frustrated and unfulfilled in life, consider *Wild Oat*.

ECZEMA*, PSORIASIS*, etc.

- *Crab Apple* helps to detox and cleanse the skin, especially if there is pus. If the skin is very red and angry *Holly* can be useful. For itchiness and irritable, nervous skin conditions use *Impatiens* or *Agrimony*. If your self-confidence suffers as a result of your skin condition, consider *Larch*. *Walnut* or *Beech* can help if you are sensitive or allergic to external influences. If there is bitterness and resentment use *Willow*. If you prefer to be on your own and have problems making contact with other people, *Water Violet* may be useful. If your skin condition recurs on a regular basis *Chestnut Bud* is best. *Gentian* helps if you feel discouraged. For all acute conditions consider *Rescue Remedy*. All Bach Remedies can also be used externally (see page 182 – The Way to Take Bach Remedies).

EXHAUSTION

See page 170 – Weakness

FATIGUE

See page 170 – Weakness

HEADACHE*/ MIGRAINE*

- This is a very good example of how many different emotional states can cause or perpetuate a physical complaint such as a headache. For tension headaches *Agrimony* can be useful, especially if you hide your worries and anxieties behind a brave face. If you feel your head is exploding, consider *Cherry Plum*. If you feel acutely stressed and overwhelmed, *Elm* is recommended. If you feel mentally exhausted, *Hornbeam* is a good choice. If your mind is spinning and you cannot shut down persistent and repetitive thoughts, take *White Chestnut*. Is there aggression or anger, or do you experience angry symptoms, such as violent, throbbing pain? If so, *Holly* is effective. If there is a lot of anger and resentment, *Willow* may be better. If you are over-enthusiastic and very committed to your beliefs, *Vervain* helps to relieve tension, strain and stress. *Oak* can be used if you push yourself beyond your limits. *Vine* helps if you are a dominating person and cannot tolerate being contradicted. Any kind of physical (e.g. whiplash) or emotional (e.g. bad news) trauma responds well to *Star of Bethlehem*. If you are very critical and intolerant of others, *Beech* is valuable. In cases where you are overcritical of yourself, take *Pine* instead. If you feel very impatient and irritable, *Impatiens* is good. For headaches and migraines which reappear periodically, *Chestnut Bud* is useful. If you experience numbness, fainting or visual disturbances prior to a migraine, *Clematis* may help. If you are bullied or neglect your own needs in order to fulfil someone else's wishes, try *Centaury*. If you cannot make up your mind and you have constantly to ask for advice, *Cerato* is appropriate. If either mentally (mood swings) or physically (vertigo, nausea) unbalanced, *Scleranthus* is useful. If you worry too much about others, *Red Chestnut* can help. Those who are stiff and inflexible (mentally or physically) need *Rock Water*.

HEARING, problems with*

- *Clematis* and *Honeysuckle* are useful if you tend to be 'deaf' to what is happening around you. *Hornbeam* is useful for those who feel mentally too tired and exhausted to be attentive. *Star of Bethlehem* is beneficial in all cases, where a shock has triggered the problem. Hearing problems in old age often correlate with arteriosclerosis or otosclerosis (page 167 – Stiffness).

IMMUNE SYSTEM, weak

See page 146 – Colds

IMPOTENCY

See page 166 – Sexual Problems

INSOMNIA*

- A very important remedy for insomnia is
White Chestnut, especially if you suffer
from an overactive mind which prevents
you from sleeping, or wakes you up early.
Aspen, *Mimulus* or *Rock Rose* are useful
for anxiety and fears of having
nightmares, of being alone, etc. *Rescue
Remedy* generally helps to calm you down
and can be combined with *Vervain*, if you
(or your child) are over-excited. If you
are desperately worried about
something, consider *Sweet Chestnut*. If
you are concerned about others, *Red
Chestnut* is useful. For anger and
resentment keep *Willow* in mind. If you
hide your worries behind a brave face,
but deep down they haunt you, take
Agrimony. If you are acutely stressed and
exhausted, consider *Elm*. You feel weak
and exhausted, but cannot sleep? Take
Olive. For insomnia and depression
consider *Mustard*. Children who tend to

be manipulative, need a lot of attention and therefore do not sleep on their own, benefit from *Chicory*. If you feel guilty about something, *Pine* is the best remedy.

MENOPAUSE, problems*

- The main remedy is *Walnut*. For mood swings and hot flushes *Scleranthus* and *Rescue Remedy* are highly recommended. For depression, consider *Mustard*. *Honeysuckle* helps if you are dwelling on the past. If there are fears, *Mimulus* is useful. For anger problems *Holly* is superb and if you fear you are losing control, *Cherry Plum* is very useful.

MIGRAINE

See page 153 – Headache

NAILS, biting

- *Agrimony* for hidden fears and anxiety, *Cherry Plum* for fear of losing control and *Impatiens* for restlessness and irritability are recommended.

OPERATION, DENTIST before and after*

- For fear (of dentists, needles, etc.) *Mimulus* is very effective. *Larch* can help with your self-confidence if you are scared. *Rescue Remedy* is a great soother of pain, tension and anxiety before and after operations. For cleansing and detox *Crab Apple* is useful. Take *Olive* and *Elm* if you feel exhausted.

OSTEOPOROSIS*, WEAK SPINE*

- Those who are weak willed and easily

exploited by others need *Centaury*. For a lack of self-confidence *Larch* is recommended.

PAIN* and INFLAMMATION*

- *Rescue Remedy* brings great relief from pain and tension and treats all kinds of minor or major emergencies, accidents and physical or emotional traumas, which can cause pain and inflammation. It contains *Rock Rose* for fear and panic, *Clematis* for keeping you conscious, *Impatiens* for irritability and tension, *Star of Bethlehem* for shock and *Cherry Plum* for the fear of losing control. These remedies have proved to be extremely valuable.

- Other remedies for pain and inflammation include: *Elm* if you feel suddenly overwhelmed by the pain; *Aspen* and *Mimulus* for fears and anxiety; *Holly* in all cases where either you feel angry or aggressive or the pain/inflammation is angry and aggressive; *Willow* for anger, bitterness and resentment causing or caused by the pain; *Beech* if the pain/inflammation becomes intolerable or makes you intolerant; *White Chestnut* if you cannot get the pain out of your mind. For recurring pains and inflammation consider *Gentian* and *Chestnut Bud*. Chronic conditions can also respond to *Wild Rose* (resignation, lack of vitality), *Gorse* (hopelessness), *Pine* (guilt complex). All kinds of inflammation respond well to *Crab Apple*.

PERIODS, problems with*

- If your period is irregular, or sometimes heavy but at other times light, take *Scleranthus*.
- For painful periods try *Rescue Remedy*.

Consider *Rock Water* if you are too hard on yourself. If you feel full of self-pity, neglected and easily hurt, take *Chicory*. If the pain is very violent and/or it makes you aggressive, *Holly* can be useful. Impatience and irritability react well to *Impatiens*. Take *Clematis* if you feel dizzy. If the pain is worse before the period starts and subsides with the bleeding or if you feel hysterical, *Cherry Plum* can be effective. If you feel highly stressed and overwhelmed by responsibilities *Elm* is a good choice. *Agrimony* helps if you tend to hide your pain and discomfort behind a brave face.

- For heavy bleeding with weakness and exhaustion consider *Olive, Elm, Wild Rose, Clematis* and *Rescue Remedy*.

PMT*

- First choose the Bach Remedies which best match the emotional problems you experience before your period. *Rescue Remedy* is helpful for anxiety and tension in general. If you feel aggressive *Holly* is the one to take. If you feel hysterical or as if you are losing control, *Cherry Plum* is extremely good. For anger and resentment take *Willow*. If you suffer from mood swings, *Scleranthus* is helpful. If there is impatience and irritability, *Impatiens* should be considered. *Mustard* helps with depression. If you feel self-pity, neglected and easily hurt take *Chicory*. Are you very intolerant and critical of others? *Beech* is helpful. If you feel unclean or you start to get very tidy, *Crab Apple* is a good choice. If you feel exhausted and tired, choose either *Hornbeam* or *Olive*. For feeling very stressed and overwhelmed *Elm* can help. If you want to be on your own, *Water Violet* is best.

PREGNANCY* and BIRTH*

- For morning sickness a combination of *Rescue Remedy, Scleranthus* (hormonal imbalance) and *Walnut* (transition) can help. Either *Mimulus* (fears), *Willow* (resentment in relation to the pregnancy) or *Hornbeam* (lack of vitality), or indeed other Bach Remedies if they suit your emotional state, can be added.

- If you feel exhausted during the later stages of the pregnancy, *Olive*, or for acute exhaustion, *Elm*, are both helpful. *Crab Apple* can help with self-disgust if you cannot accept your body. For increasing nervousness and tension *Rescue Remedy* is recommended. If you are over-anxious about the baby, consider *Red Chestnut*.

- When giving birth *Rescue Remedy* has often proved to be extremely helpful. *Elm* and *Olive* can help to give you strength. *Walnut* again helps with the transition.

- After giving birth *Olive* can help you if you feel completely exhausted. *Mimulus* helps with fears. Take *Elm* if you feel overwhelmed by these new responsibilities, *Larch* if you lack self-confidence, *Sweet Chestnut* for complete desperation, *Mustard* for depression and/or *Red Chestnut* if you worry too much about the baby. *Walnut* is again useful for the transition.

PSORIASIS

See page 152 – Eczema

RESTLESSNESS*, NERVOUSNESS

- If you hide your worries and anxieties behind a brave face, *Agrimony* is recommended. Do you feel as if you are losing control? In this case *Cherry Plum* is a useful remedy. If you are indecisive and you constantly ask others for advice, take *Cerato*. For impatience and irritability use *Impatiens*. *Mimulus* is helpful if you are shy, timid, fearful and blush easily. Take *Red Chestnut* if the worrying over others makes you restless and nervous. For over-activity and over-enthusiasm *Vervain* is a good choice.

SEXUAL PROBLEMS*, such as IMPOTENCY*, AVERSION to sex, etc.

- If fears are a problem (such as the fear of not being able to perform, of pregnancy, disease) *Mimulus* is a good choice. For a lack of self-confidence choose *Larch*. If you have bad experiences, *Star of Bethlehem* can help. If there is a moral or guilt issue, *Pine* is recommended. For disgust (e.g. of sex and bodily fluids) or self-disgust take *Crab Apple*. For over-excitement consider *Vervain* and *Impatiens*. For physical weakness (e.g. for impotency) or exhaustion try *Olive*.

SPINE, weak

See page 159 – Osteoporosis

STIFFNESS* (including arteriosclerosis)

- *Rock Water* is the main remedy for mental and physical inflexibility and stiffness. *Oak* is recommended if you push yourself beyond your limits, if you are stubborn, inflexible and unrelenting with yourself. *Vine* is a useful remedy if you cannot accept contradiction and have a tendency to dominate others.

Water Violet is the right choice for those who are shy, independent and prefer to be on their own. *Star of Bethlehem* is beneficial in all cases where shock or trauma has caused the stiffness. Stiffness can also be caused by stress (see page 128).

TEETH, grinding

• *Agrimony* is useful if you hide your worries and anxieties behind a brave face. An overactive mind which will not let you relax can be treated with *White Chestnut*. If you push yourself too hard, *Oak* can be useful. *Vervain* helps with over-activity. Anger and resentment respond well to *Holly* or *Willow*.

TRAVEL SICKNESS*

• The Bach Remedy to try is *Scleranthus*.

VISION, problems with*

- *Clematis* and *Honeysuckle* are useful if you tend not to be interested in the present, or if you spend too much time looking at a TV or computer screen. *Clematis* (with *Olive*) is also useful for blurred vision, caused by low blood pressure and weakness. *Hornbeam* is helpful for those who feel mentally fatigued, have tired eyes and become short-sighted. *Star of Bethlehem* is beneficial in all cases where a shock has caused the problem. Stress (see page 128) is often responsible for many visual problems. Cataracts are a kind of stiffness (see page 167) of the lens. All the remedies can be used externally as a compress. (See page 182 – The *Way to Take* Bach Remedies)

WEAKNESS*, FATIGUE*, EXHAUSTION*

- The main remedy for physical and mental fatigue and exhaustion is *Olive*. If you are overwhelmed by responsibilities and stress, *Elm* is recommended. *Clematis* is useful if you lack energy and feel faint. If you have pushed yourself beyond your limits and still do not allow yourself to rest, *Oak* should be used. Are you exhausted because you give too much of yourself to others? In such cases *Centaury* is the best. Do you feel insecure and constantly change your mind? Then *Cerato* is preferable. If you feel depressed and fatigued, consider *Mustard*. If you feel apathetic, lack energy and have given up all hope of getting better, *Wild Rose* is helpful. Should you blame yourself constantly and push yourself hard, try *Pine*. If you are over-enthusiastic in your approach and over-exert yourself in the name of your ideals, take *Vervain*. If you cannot shut down your mind, and have persistent, repetitive thoughts which cause insomnia and exhaustion, *White Chestnut* is worth trying.

WEATHER, sensitive to changes

- *Rescue Remedy* often has a beneficial effect if you suffer acutely from changes in the weather. Another important Bach Remedy is *Scleranthus*. If you feel irritable, consider *Holly*, if you are tired *Hornbeam*, suddenly exhausted *Elm*, or if depressed *Mustard*.

REMEDIES FOR CHILDREN AND BABIES

Children often respond extremely well to Bach Remedies which help to harmonize their behaviour and support their development. However, as it is not easy for children to answer so many questions, you have to rely more upon close, accurate observation. This can at times make it more difficult to select the right remedy. Generally speaking, all the recommendations in this book can be used to treat children, but in this chapter you will find some advice specific to children and babies.

It is worth remembering that the behaviour of children can be strongly influenced by the way in which their parents or siblings treat them. The family dynamic is also significant. In some cases it may be helpful if both parents and child take Bach Remedies.

Always be aware of the limitations of self-treatment. See page 182 – When should you seek professional help?

Bedwetting

- For the fear of losing control give *Cherry Plum* and *Mimulus*. For feeling guilty consider *Pine*. If bedwetting is used as a means of getting attention or to manipulate, *Chicory* can produce very good results. If the child is resentful and sulky, *Willow* is preferable.

Examinations, fear of

- For acute fear just before or even during an exam, *Rescue Remedy* should be taken and kept close at hand.

- If afraid that they will not pass, give *Mimulus*.
- For acute exhaustion and stress, try *Elm*.
- For a lack of self-confidence, *Larch* is very effective.
- If your child constantly asks others for advice or feels insecure and corrects the things he has actually done right, *Cerato* should be added.
- Consider *Gentian* if there is pessimism and discouragement.
- For children who strive and are over-ambitious, *Rock Water* is a good choice.
- For the shock of a previous negative examination experience *Star of Bethlehem* and *Honeysuckle* should be considered.

Homesickness

See page 106 – Homesickness

Hyperactivity

- If the child always seems to be rushing around, try *Impatiens*. This is the main remedy for hyperactivity.
- If your child is over-enthusiastic about something and cannot settle down, *Vervain* is useful.
- If your child keeps jumping from one activity to another use *Scleranthus* and *Wild Oat*.
- *Rescue Remedy* helps to relax and to calm children down.

Learning difficulties

- The main remedy for learning difficulties is *Chestnut Bud*. If your child lacks self-confidence, *Larch* should be considered first. If your child constantly asks others for advice or feels insecure and corrects the things he has actually done right, *Cerato* should be added. Also give *Gentian*

if your child is easily discouraged. For a
lack of motivation *Wild Rose* is helpful.
For a lack of energy choose either
Hornbeam or *Olive*.

- For a lack of concentration see page 92.
- For forgetfulness see page 103.

Restless, sleepless babies

- If due to some trauma or shock (e.g.
  birth), the symptoms will respond well to
  Star of Bethlehem.
- Are fears (e.g. of being alone or the
  darkness) and nightmares the reason for
  the restlessness? If so, *Aspen*, *Mimulus* or
  Rock Rose are useful in such cases.
- For impatience and restlessness, add
  Impatiens.
- For an overactive mind, add *White
  Chestnut*.
- If your child always seeks attention and

tries to manipulate you, *Chicory* is helpful.

- If there is a lot of angry shouting, *Holly* is the best remedy.
- If your child cries desperately, *Sweet Chestnut* is preferable.
- For teething see below.

Restlessness, aggressive behaviour, temper tantrums

- For children who lose control, have temper tantrums and are suddenly violent, *Cherry Plum* or *Rescue Remedy* are helpful.
- For anger problems *Holly* is best.
- If the child does a lot of bullying, does not listen to authority and hates to be contradicted, *Vine* will be good.
- For restless and impatient behaviour use *Impatiens*.

- *Chicory* is the best remedy if children are demanding and in need of constant attention.
- If your child is going through a transition such as teething, puberty, the arrival of a new sibling, starting school, moving house, etc., add *Walnut*.

Teething

- The main remedy for teething is *Walnut*.
- If the child seems irritable and restless, add *Impatiens*. If moody and aggressive, add *Holly*. If weepy and clingy, add *Chicory*.
- For teething pain mix *Cherry Plum*, *Elm* and *White Chestnut*. See also page 160 – Pain.

THE TREATMENT OF ANIMALS AND PLANTS

Both animals and plants respond very well to treatment with Bach Remedies. This only confirms their effectiveness, because a placebo effect surely cannot take place when nursing a plant. Treat animals and plants in the same way as human beings.

Animals

If the animal shows signs of fear, aggression, lack of interest, etc., treat it as indicated in the chapters on Emotional and Physical Complaints from A to Z. For all cases of shock, accidents, injuries, pre- and post-surgical work, *Rescue Remedy* has proved to be extremely effective.

Plants

For uprooting, or other shocking events in a plant's life, give *Rescue Remedy* or *Star of Bethlehem* (even freshly cut flowers will last longer). If the plant looks exhausted or weak, consider *Olive* or *Hornbeam*. Infested plants may benefit from *Crab Apple*.

PART
FIVE

THE WAY TO TAKE BACH REMEDIES

Internal use of Bach Remedies

A (= acute):

If you suffer from an acute problem use 3 drops of each of the chosen remedies to half a glass of water, mix it well and take a few sips from it at least four times a day.

C (= chronic):

If your problems have existed for quite some time add 3 drops of each appropriate remedy to an empty 30ml (1oz) dropper bottle (available from most Bach Remedy distributors and chemists – see also Useful Addresses on page 190) and fill the bottle up with still mineral or spring water. Shake it well. Take 5 drops of this mixture at least four times a day for several weeks.

To avoid any interference with the effect of the remedy you should not eat, drink or brush your teeth five minutes before and after taking it. Keep the liquid in your mouth for a few seconds.

External use of Bach Remedies

As a compress:
This can help against tension, light burns, skin irritation and inflammation and tired eyes. For the compress add 6 drops of the selected remedy to half a litre (1 pint) of clean water. Wet a cloth or flannel and

hold next to the skin. For inflamation a cool cloth is best, for other complaints use a warm cloth. Repeat whenever needed.

In the bath:

This can help with tension, skin problems, etc. Put 12 drops of the stock bottle or 20 drops of the ready-made mixture (see B) into your bath. Repeat every one to seven days.

The use of Bach Rescue Cream is explained on page 14 (*Rescue Remedy*).

HOW TO STORE THE REMEDIES

Bach Remedy stock bottles should be stored in a dark place at room temperature, away from strong smelling substances (such as perfumes or essential oils) and kept out of the reach of children. Stored in this way they will last for years.

In personally-made mixtures, the water can go off after some weeks, especially in the summer. To avoid this you can add 10ml ($1/3$ of the dropper bottle) of brandy or cider vinegar when you mix your remedies. Alternatively store the 30-ml dropper bottle in the fridge. Stop using the mixture if there is a change of colour or taste.

POSSIBLE REACTIONS AFTER TAKING BACH REMEDIES

The remedies work

In this case your condition improves. Often one feels an initial uplifting feeling, followed by the improvement of the physical complaints. As a rule acute problems respond more quickly to the right remedy. Very often you will feel an improvement within the first three to four weeks. Less acute and chronic problems and conditions can take longer (several weeks or months).

The remedies don't work/no longer work

If you don't feel better after four to six weeks you may have chosen the wrong remedies, so check the choice of remedies and try to find more appropriate ones. Be aware that during a treatment your situation may change and different remedies might become more helpful. Be aware that the use of antidepressants and similar drugs may slow down or diminish the effect of Bach Remedies.

Side-effects and risks?

Bach Remedies have no known side-effects or negative interactions with any other medication. They can safely be used to treat children, adults and even pregnant women.

Bach Remedies can be combined with any kind of other treatment. They can support other therapies – conventional or complementary. Please tell your homeopath or other practitioner that you intend to use Bach Remedies.

There is only one risk with this form of self-treatment: this does not come from the remedies themselves but from the possible delay which can occur before the right remedies are identified and taken. If your condition does not improve, seek professional help sooner rather than later!

When should you seek professional help?

The Little Book of Bach Flower Remedies recommends self-treatment only for common and minor problems and complaints, for which you would not normally seek immediate help from your GP or a psychologist/psychotherapist.

Generally speaking you should always see your GP, a psychologist/psychotherapist or an experienced Bach practitioner if:

- the condition/symptoms is/are severe, very acute or unusual
- your condition does not improve or even gets worse
- you feel at all unsure about self-treatment
- conditions have already existed for some time, are chronic or frequently recur.

But you can safely take Bach Remedies alongside other, prescribed medication or treatment.

USEFUL ADDRESSES

For further information about Bach practi-
tioners or other advice contact:

Dr Edward Bach Centre, Mount Vernon,
Bakers Lane, Sotwell, Oxfordshire,
OX10 0PZ, UK
Tel. 01491 834678
email: bach@bachcentre.com
website: www. bachcentre.com

Helios Pharmacy prepares Bach Remedy
mixtures on individual demand. They use
the Healing Herbs range of Bach
Remedies. Contact:

89-97 Camden Road, Tunbridge Wells,
Kent, TN1 2QR.
Tel: 01892 537254/536393
email: pharmacy@helios.co.uk
website: www.helios.co.uk

The distributor of Bach Flower Remedies
is A. Nelson & Co., Broadheath House,
83 Parkside, London, SW19 5LP, UK.

The distributor of the Healing Herbs of
Dr Edward Bach is Healing Herbs Ltd,
P.O. Box 65, Hereford, HR2 0UW, UK.

Recommended Reading

Bach Edward, *Heal Thyself*, The C.W.
   Daniel Company

Weeks Nora and Bullen Victor, *The Bach
   Flower Remedies*, The C.W. Daniel
   Company

Chancellor Philip M., *Handbook of the Bach
   Flower Remedies*, The C.W. Daniel
   Company

Scheffer Mechthild, *Bach Flower Therapy*,
   HarperCollins

Blome Gotz, *Advanced Bach Flower Therapy*,
   Healing Arts Press

ABOUT THE AUTHOR

Sven Sommer trained in Bach Flower
Therapy and other complementary
therapies in Germany. He is the author
of six books, including *The Little Book of
Homeopathy*. Since 1997 he has worked
and lived in Oxford. For more
information you can visit his website:
www.svensommer.com